The Power of Habits

Change your thoughts change your life live in happiness.

Description

While change is something that is always on many people's minds, the number of individuals who follow through on the changes they envision for themselves are relatively few and far between. This all comes down to the truth of the matter which is that, while random change is easy, true, meaningful change can be extremely tricky to get just right. If you are ready to stop thinking about making a change and to actually get to work doing it then *The Power of Habits Change your thoughts change your life live in happiness* is the book that you have been waiting for.

True change can only ever come from within as external factors alone can never be enough to generate the level of drive that long-lasting change requires. As such, if you ever hope to see long change then the first thing that you are going to need to do is ensure you have the right tools for the job. This is why this book not only discusses how to set the types of goals and create personal patterns that lead to the types of change you are looking for, it tells you how exactly to go about doing so, starting with ensuring that you have the right type of mindset to maximize change in a minimal period of time. You will also learn how confidence and discipline come together to make the type of change you are dreaming about a reality sooner than you might realize.

It doesn't matter how far-fetched the long-term changes that you want to make may seem right now, if you break it down into realistic chunks them you will be surprised at how quickly you can actually turn your dreams into reality. While the first goal that you are planning to set might not seem like much at the moment, the truth of the matter is that it is akin to the acorn that can grow into the mighty oak tree. If you persevere now and see your first goal through to the end, then that will start to create the types of neural pathways that will eventually lead to positive patterns and positive habits that could very well last the rest of your life. So, what are you waiting for? Get ready to make long lasting changes and buy this book today!

Inside you will find

- How to tell if you have a fixed or growth mindset and what that means for your propensity for change.
- The best way to improve your self-discipline levels no matter what type of change you are hoping to cultivate.
- Why confidence and change go hand in hand and how to improve the former to enhance the latter.
- Positive personal patterns to be on the lookout for and those to avoid at all costs.
- The best way to set the best goals to achieve your dreams.
- *And more...*

Table of Contents

Introduction

Congratulations on downloading *The Power of Habits Change your thoughts change your life live in happiness* and thank you for doing so. While change is something that is always on many people's minds, the number of individuals who follow through on the changes they envision for themselves are relatively few and far between. This all comes down to the truth of the matter which is that, while random change is easy, true, meaningful change can be extremely tricky to get just right.

Luckily, there are numerous different ways you can make attracting the right types of change into your life, while not necessarily easier, certainly much more attainable which is why the following chapters will discuss everything you can do to help ensure that change works with you, not against you. The first thing you need to know to ensure you make major change as easy on yourself as possible is the type of mindset you currently approach challenges with, there are two separate and distinct options and one is much more certain to set you up for success than the other.

Next you will learn how important it is to remain disciplined while you are looking to cultivate major change in your life as no change ever came about overnight. With that out of the way you will learn all about the many ways confidence factors into true personal change and how to improve one to enhance your chance of the other. Then you will learn all about cultivating personal patterns and finally you will learn all about setting the right type of goals to find the success you seek.

There are plenty of books on this subject on the market, thanks again for choosing this one! Every effort was made to ensure it is full of as much useful information as possible, please enjoy!

Chapter 1: Understand Your Current Mindset

True change can only ever come from within as external factors alone can never be enough to generate the level of drive that long-lasting change requires. As such, if you ever hope to see long change then the first thing that you are going to need to do is ensure you have the right type of mindset for the job. To understand a truly pro-change mindset, the first thing that you are going to want to do is to ask yourself why it is that some individuals seem to fall backwards into success while others can only ever seem to fall short no matter how hard they try even though they seem just as skilled as those for whom success comes easily. The answer is that the successful person believed in themselves and their abilities, it is as simple as that.

Polarizing mindsets
The ease with which you are able to successfully make the decision to change, and stick with that change in the long term, likely stems from the way that you perceive your most prized skills and talents and has no doubt been the same since your earliest memories. While they likely had no idea what it is that they were doing, at some point someone either praised you for how hard you tried in order to achieve something or for how naturally gifted you were to achieve your success. If you were praised for your hard work, then you learned that hard work equates with success; while if you were praised for your natural talents then you likely learned they were innate and could not be changed. The first scenario is what is known as the growth mindset while the second is known as a fixed mindset and should be avoided at all costs if you ever hope to successfully change for the better.

Overall, the growth oriented mindset is one that always appreciates criticism that is given in a constructive fashion and finds success in others inspiring instead of threatening. Furthermore, this feeling of inspiration extends to all obstacles they find in their path as they are more likely to see them as learning experiences rather than reasons to give up which means they always appreciate a challenge no matter how steep. This is a natural side effect of their long-term focus and belief that success is not possible without serious effort.

On the other hand, those with a fixed mindset are unlikely to listen to feedback, regardless of how well-meaning its intent, because they find success in others to be extremely threatening regardless of the venue where it is expressed. This is because they believe that success is only innate which makes them naturally want to avoid challenge and give up when presented with obstacles that would require personal growth while at the same time ensuring that they appear as competent as possible at all times. While it is clear why the pair of mindsets would ultimately diverge so significantly, it is also important to keep in mind that they both ultimately germinate from the same, perfectly natural act of receiving praise for a job well done.

Based on the type of praise that they receive, children's brains ultimately learn to either receive pleasure from being told they are successful (those with a fixed mindset) or from actually succeeding against an existing challenge (those with a growth mindset). One side of this dichotomy or the other is almost guaranteed to be a part of each and every person's personality, and if you find it difficult to get over how others see you, then there is a good chance that you fall on the fixed, versus the growth, side of things. On the contrary, if you find it relatively easy to look within and find the extra bit of strength you need to preserve and make positive changes then you likely already have a growth mindset and will likely benefit more from other chapters in this book.

It is important to try and circumvent your fixed mindset whenever possible as in addition to reacting to positive experience differently, they also react differently to negative experiences as well. Specifically, those who find themselves burdened with a fixed mindset will find even somewhat minor setbacks towards their current goal as a reason to give up on the entire endeavor entirely. This is caused by the core belief that they will never have more tools to defeat the obstacle than they do in the moment so trying multiple times is akin to the definition of madness because nothing will ever change, period.

It shouldn't be difficult to understand why this reductive thinking can easily turn a minor roadblock into an impassable barrier and why it can make it difficult to start even relatively simple projects. This is exactly what makes the growth mindset to the process of personal change, those with a growth mindset are sure to always appreciate a good challenge.

Changing your mindset

By this point it should be obvious to you whether you have a growth or a fixed mindset and why it is so important to prioritize the one above the other. Luckily, in this case knowing really is half the battle as it is only by knowing that you are burdened with a fixed mindset that you can start making real progress towards changing it for the better. As luck would have it, the human brain changes noticeably and visibly throughout its lifespan, based on the stimuli that it receives on a regular basis. As such, it doesn't matter how deeply seated a given idea, trait or characteristic is, given enough of the proper stimuli there is nothing that cannot be overwritten.

At its most basic, the human brain functions as neurons travel along preexisting neural pathways taking a path of least resistance to ensure that thoughts move as quickly as possible. As new neural pathways are formed, they are worn-in with use which means that in order to change from a fixed to a growth mindset all you need to do is to commit to practice growth mindset inducing behaviors as frequently as possible. This doesn't mean the process is going to be easy, however, as unfortunately the fixed mindset pathways are going to be some of the most well-worn of them all. It will be possible, however, and that possibility is what you are going to need to hang on too as tightly as you can and use that thought as a lifeline when your natural inclination to give up kicks in. In addition to holding on to the possibility of change, you may find the following tips useful when it comes to permanently changing your mindset for the better.

Go all in: As previously mentioned, there are few core assumptions that your mind makes that run deeper than your fixed mindset. As such, in order to ensure that you don't waste an undue amount of time fighting that uphill battle only to quit 30 days down the line, the first thing that you will want to do is to commit yourself fully to the task at hand. True change will never happen without a growth mindset, it really is key to the entire process which means you are going to need to commit fully to the alterations you are striving for if you ever want to see change in any specific areas of your life. When you start out, it is important that you consider the fact that altering your mental state is a marathon, not a sprint, which means that slow and steady wins the race. Take things slow and don't expect results overnight if you ever hope to find real success.

Start small: In order to permanently change your neural pathways for the better, the first thing that you will need to do is to set a manageable goal that you only have to step outside your comfort zone a small amount to reach. Once you succeed and achieve your goal, you will then be able to look back on that moment in the future when the going has started actually getting tough and use the fact that perseverance equaled success previously to give yourself the mental boost required to push forward no matter what the task at hand. Furthermore, it is important to keep in mind the cumulative effect that each and every action based on growth mindset principles you take has on your mindset as a whole. While one or two small actions won't be enough to sway things, enough of those small actions pooled together will start to stack up. Keep putting one foot in front of the other and you will be surprised by the results.

Look back on every day: While you are first starting out, you will likely find that you have difficultly retaining a burgeoning growth mindset as the day wears on. If this is the case, you will likely find it helpful to keep a ledger tallying all of your growth and fixed mindset thoughts throughout the day. Simply keep track of each and pay special attention to the period of time that typifies a transition from positive to negative. While this may simply be a case of the day wearing on you, it may also be related to a specific event which you are not even aware of. The only way you will know is if you map it all out in front of yourself every day for at least a month to provide you will all the data that you need to make an informed decision.

Have realistic expectations: Finally, you are going to want to keep in mind the fact that just because someone has a growth mindset doesn't mean that they are going to be happy about everything negative that befalls them. After all, everyone is simply going to have a bad day now and then; the important thing to remember is that while everyone might have an urge to give up when the going gets tough, those who have a growth mindset manage to ignore this feeling and preserve until they find the success that they have been searching for. It is important to compartmentalize these feelings rather than letting them dangerously spiral to the point that they are much more difficult to ignore than they might otherwise be. Don't let a moment of doubt turn into a day, hour or even a minute, commit to change and find the growth mindset hiding inside you right now.

Chapter 2: The Importance of Discipline

While it might seem hard to comprehend, the fact of the matter is that those who are committed to changing their lives in a positive fashion are prone to feeling just as lethargic, angst-ridden or depressed as everyone else. If this is the case, then the only difference between them and everyone else is that they have the personal discipline to stop those feelings in their tracks and make the hard choices they need to in order to improve their current situation. While ensuring that you have the proper type of mindset to help you find the change you are looking for, ensuring that you have the proper self-discipline to follow through when the going gets tough will make it easier for you to make the changes you want and stick with them in the long term.

In addition to helping you meet change in the most effective way possible, you will be pleased to learn that being self-disciplined also has numerous ancillary benefits that are sure to help you approach your path to change in the most effective manner possible. Specifically, it will help you to follow through on your goals more easily while at the same time making it easier to choose realistic goals you can set for yourself to follow through on in both the short and the long term. Regardless of the goals you choose, self-discipline will surely be a positive force in your life that will never dessert you regardless of the insurmountable odds ahead of you. What's more, it can make it much easier to disregard distraction and ignore temptation even when it is staring you in the face. Get started boosting your self-discipline with the following tips.

Be patient: Being self-disciplined means you will always take the time to completely understand whatever it is you are currently working towards to ensure you are attacking it from the most productive angle possible. Remember, the more potential issues you are aware of when it comes to the current goal, the more easily you will be able to nip them in the bud and ensure that they do not do more harm than that which is completely unavoidable. When it comes to understanding your desire for personal change, this means looking deep within yourself and figuring out just what is holding you back so that you can get to the root of the matter and get things sorted as soon as possible.

Know when to act: Learning to enhance your self-discipline means understanding that it is better to gather your resources and move when the time is right rather than pressing forward blindly. Just as it is important to do research in order to determine the best course of action for your goals, it is equally important to know when it is actually time to stop worrying about gathering data and start worrying about acting on what has already been gathered. In your quest for personal change you are likely going to find issues and shortcomings that you will have difficultly coming at head on. It is important to stay the course when this occurs, however, as being self-disciplined means pushing forward for the greater good no matter what. Remember, self-discipline is a skill and like any skill it will only improve as you practice it; what's more, each time you do will make the next time you are required to that much easier.

Act in the right way: While actually taking the action might seem self-explanatory, the truth of the matter is that all action can be split into implementation as well as completion. Completion involves acting on an existing plan and following through on any goals that you may be currently working towards which means it is crucial to ensuring that you use self-discipline in the right way, every time. Implementation involves determining the plan that is optimal for the situation based on the research that you have already completed.

Committing to being disciplined

When it comes to your journey to discover your internal ability to make real, lasting change, it is perfectly natural to find building your level of self-discipline more difficult than you might realistically prefer, especially if you are working on adopting a growth mindset at the same time. One way to actively move the process along in the proper direction is too commit whole-hog to a major long-term goal that will both improve your life in a noticeable way and require a great deal of self-discipline in order to completely successfully at the same time. This could be anything from finishing that musical you have always dreamed of writing to getting in shape and staying there, the specifics don't matter all that does is starting something that will help you get in the habit of practicing self-discipline on the regular.

Taking on this task should be somewhat scary, and it is perfectly acceptable if you don't have the end clearly in sight just yet. The fact of the matter is that simply by undertaking the task in question will help you begin to improve your baseline level of self-discipline while also giving you something to focus on beside your specific desire to change, allowing you to work on changing indirectly as well. When it comes to choosing the right task for the job the first thing that you will want to do is consider the types of triggers and negative influences that you currently find make it easy for you to slip back into negative habits and patterns that you are currently trying to avoid. Knowing what causes you to revert to negative behavior is the first step to preventing it in the future as it will help you become more aware of the common excuses you use as a way of validating behaviors you are really better off avoiding.

Choosing the right project is an important consideration as jumping in to the wrong projection without the right preparations is only going to lead to disaster which will make it even more difficult for you to get started the next time around because you will have a whole new list of reasons for not getting started right this minute. As such, the best choice is to pick something that is difficult enough that you will have to exert willpower in order to achieve it while not being so major that it will take something close to an act of god in order to make it a reality. While you might be on a roll when it comes to making positive self-changes, it is important to not expect too much too soon in order to achieve the best results.

When it comes time to implement new self-discipline focused habits into your daily routines, you are going to want to break them down into bite-sized chunks that can be slipped into existing routines for the best success. Making them part of existing habits will cause them to switch from being something new to something old hat almost overnight which is important as improving your self-discipline is only something that will happen if you work at it diligently every single day. If you do so, you will find that over time you will slowly develop the ability to make and maintain the type of change that you have been looking for.

Don't be afraid to burn your ship

When the Spanish conquistadors first landed in South America, the man in charge, Hernan Cortez, made the apparently rash decision of burning his fleet of ships while his men watched from the foreign shore. Despite this seemingly mad decision, Cortez had, in fact, made an acute judgement of the situation and determined that this was the only way that he was ever going to ensure that his men were committed enough to the task ahead of them to take this foreign land from the natives. While such a task wouldn't regularly require those types of extreme measures, Cortez's men were sick and tired from their journey and he knew that making sure that they knew they had no other options was the only way that they were going to find success.

The understanding that the only options were success or death served to motivate Cortez's men in the anticipated fashion and you can use this same process to motivate yourself to help get into the habit of taking self-disciplined action whenever the opportunity presents itself. You will find this especially effective when you are interested in working up to more complicated goals or those that you feel as though they are within your reach, but only just. Before you have fully formed the most effective habits for success you may find that get sidetracked on occasion despite your best intentions, making a habit of burning your bridges can help you to find the focus that you need in order to put your nose to the grindstone.

Cut your safety net: Remember, self-discipline is not something that you can call into play only when you feel the need, it is either on or off, there is no in between. When you are working on building this habit it is common to find that the brain feels a need to prioritize activities that provide instant gratification, especially if the goal you are working towards seems more abstract or if there is not already a penalty for failure in place. This is when taking the extra step to remove your safety net can be especially effective as you will then have no choice but to push forward no matter how tough the going gets in the interim. It works by removing the choice from the situation, you literally have no choice but to succeed.

As an example, consider when you are working on a major project for your job, if you are struggling to meet a tight deadline go ahead and schedule the big meeting to show off your progress before you are quite sure that you can finish it. The understanding that there is no wiggle room when it comes to your success or failure will make it much more difficult for your brain to manufacture excuses and focus on getting the job done. Don't forget, those who are self-disciplined don't need to worry about plan B because such a thing is for people who are unsure if they have the follow through to complete their original plan without fail.

As you move closer to the deadline you will find that you are naturally inclined to work more and more rigorously as the anxiety of the impeding deadline mounts. This anxiety can be used in your favor as well as you will find that removing it through additional hard work and preparation is enough of a motivation to keep you working hard even when the going gets tough. With any luck, eventually you will be able to connect a pattern of self-discipline with one of stress reduction and following through in this fashion will become second nature.

Once you find yourself able to reliably burn your bridges in a professional setting the next thing that you will want to do is apply that same mentality to your personal goals as well. This can be easier said than done, however, as it can be difficult to create the same type of urgency when there isn't anyone standing over your head providing you with the adequate amount of motivation you need to make you really not want to fail. The best option in this case is typically going to be looking for external motivation in the form of a social circle or club that is dedicated to the same general goal that you are currently working towards.

You will be surprised how effective an external source of motivation can be when it comes to cutting the excuses out of the equation and helping you to get to the heart of the matter time after time. If there isn't a readily available group that you can turn to with your goal, at the very least you should reach out to a friend or loved one to help you remain accountable to the end result that you determine will be enough to help you stop dreaming about reaching your goals and start actually doing it.

Chapter 3: The Importance of Confidence

When it comes to finding the will to implement true change in the long term, you will find that having confidence in yourself comes part and parcel with meeting any goals you set for yourself. If you are someone who has never had much self-confidence, then you will no doubt be surprised to learn that anyone you envy for their self-confidence was once in the exact same situation that you now find yourself in, the only difference between where they are now versus then is that they made a concentrated effort to boost their self-confidence, bit by bit, one day at a time.

This is good news for those who are interested in improving their self-confidence levels as it means that all that you need to do in order to believe in yourself more thoroughly is practice believing in yourself more regularly. Once you have the self-confidence you need to really believe that you can do anything, then making the deep down personal changes that you are aiming for can't be far behind. Boosting your confidence is something that can be done practically any time and any place, keep the following in mind moving forward and you will find your attitude towards your current level of self-confidence changing without you even realizing it.

Consider where your fears come from

When they find themselves about to be confronted with a scenario where they would ideally be able to present a self-confident self-image to those around them, the first thing that goes through many people's minds is fear. This is a response that is only ever going to do you more harm than good, however, which is why it is in your best interest to do as much as you can to change this mentality for one that is more beneficial by trying the following tips.

Reframe the situation: When you are next presented with an instance where anxiety or fright are making it difficult for you to face the situation you currently find yourself in head on, you may find success by reframing the situation so that instead of being afraid you can be curious instead. You may find success by treating the oncoming instance as something of a learning experience when it comes to changing for the better and improving your overall level of self-confidence in the process. While it might seem far-fetched, the truth of the matter is that trading fear for curiosity can make many interactions proceed much more smoothly than they otherwise might.

Seek out the root of the issue: The next time that you find yourself becoming afraid at the thought of an upcoming situation that requires self-confidence, you may find it helpful to instead consider just what it is about the situation in question that has left you feeling so afraid. While you might think the answer is obvious at first, apart from the occasional situation where fear is valid, nine times out of ten you will find that there is much less to fear than you may have originally thought. With only a small amount of rational consideration you will likely find that the truth of the situation you currently find yourself in is much less severe than any of the worst-case scenarios that you have dreamt up in your head. With this exercise completed you will then find that it is much easier to approach the current situation with a calm mind and a confident attitude.

Make a noted effort to change: In the moments where you are having an extremely hard time getting over the hump of your own insecurities and projecting confidence to the fullest degree possible, instead of wallowing in doubt, consider using these moments as a powerful catalyst for change. What could be more different in the moment than acting confident instead of worrying about what you lack? From there, that success will make it easier for a repeat performance and so on and so forth.

Know when to act: Getting to the root of your fears is important, but only in as much as it will help you act in the moment. Much like with the bigger changes you are looking to make, gathering up the self-confidence required to act is important, but only as long as the process doesn't take so long that the moment has passed once you actually find the courage to do what needs to be done. Being confident doesn't mean acting without thinking, it simply means planning with confidence in yourself and then translating those plans into actions.

Be aware of your strengths and weaknesses

If you are ever going to be confident in yourself enough to change for the better, you are going to need to look within and have a frank discussion with yourself about what you find. This means taking an honest look at not just your strengths, but all your flaws and weaknesses as well. While it might seem rather basic, the reality of the situation is that a solid round of self-analysis will do you some good, no matter what type of larger changes you are looking to make.

The best way to get started knowing yourself more intimately is to find a large mirror somewhere private and then stand in front of it completely naked. While many people will no doubt consider this a literal version of torture, persevering through the initial moments of discomfort is sure to lead to a number of surprising revelations. First and foremost, among them is that you likely don't look nearly as bad as the mental picture that you have in your head might indicate. The reality might very well be worse in some situations, but likely better in others as well. Regardless, the only way you can ever expect to mount a charge for change is by knowing exactly where you need to launch the first attack.

When it comes to making changes that are sure to boost your confidence levels, you will want to start with areas that are going to cause you to see the greatest overall difference in the shortest period of time possible. This may mean cutting back on a few troubling foods or it could be the start of a major dietary and exercise trend, the specifics don't matter, what does is that you make a concentrated effort to change and stick with it in the long term. Even if you are lucky enough to only need to tighten things up a little bit, make a point of going out and getting a nice haircut or buying some new clothes, making an effort at this stage is a key part of making any future changes stick.

Be appropriately assertive

Once you start to approach life in a more confident fashion, it will naturally assert itself as part of your day to day interactions. While this is certainly an understandable extension of all of the work you are doing, it is important to not overdo it by taking advantage of those who have not yet learned that confidence is merely a state of mind. Specifically, it is important to be seen as being assertive, without crossing over the line into actively being aggressive which is why you will want to be aware of the verbal and physical expressions you use when speaking your mind to ensure you properly walk the line between confidence and arrogance. Be mindful of the ways in which you assert yourself by keeping the following tips in mind the next time you head out into the world.

Know when to speak up: While you are still working on establishing a baseline level of self-confidence in social situations one of the best ways to go about doing so is by making a habit of sticking up for yourself when you feel as though you are getting the short end of the stick. If you don't stand up for yourself when the opportunity arises then you are essentially giving anyone that witnesses the initial incident a free pass to walk all over you as you are not important enough to warrant an extension of basic respect.

What's worse, this will only reinforce the types of negative habits that you are no doubt working so very hard to change. Specifically, things like changing yourself for others and seeking external approval instead of working to be happy with yourself and who you are personally are both common traps that those without self-confidence fall into. Rather than making you seem confrontational, standing up for yourself is a great way to show those around you that you value your time and your opinions and that they should show you the courtesy of doing the same.

Be prepared: When it comes to making the actual move to be assertive in a given situation you are always going to want to take an extra moment to prepare beforehand as you only have one opportunity to get things right. Specifically, you are going to want to start off by looking at the current situation objectively and ensuring that you are in the right before making a scene. Nothing will deflate your argument faster than finding out the facts are not on your side and it will make it more difficult for you to assert yourself in the future besides.

With knowledge that right, and common courtesy, are on your side you will then want to move forward with a clear solution to the current issue as you will find that the situation is much more likely to favorably resolve itself if you have clear plan in place for doing so. Once you know what it is that you are going to say, the next thing that you will want to do is to approach the other party using plenty of authoritative body language. This means you will want to walk with a straight back and your head held high. When you stand in front of the other person you are going to want to square your feet and your shoulders and let your arms naturally hang at your sides. When you speak, make sure to make eye contact with the other person and avoid crossing your arms at all costs as this is often considered a sign of weakness.

Speak your mind: When you do talk to the other party you are going to want to ensure that you use a voice that is calm but still authoritative and a little bit quitter than your normal speaking voice. Making the other person strain to hear you is a power play as it means they automatically have to let you control the situation in order to know what is going on. The tone that you use is extremely important as it needs to make the other person believe that obeying you is the logical choice of action. Making it clear to other people that you are confident is all about letting them know that you are in control of the current situation. When you start speaking you want to make it clear what your issue is and then follow up directly with how you plan to rectify it so the conversation starts with all the elements clearly laid on the table.

During this discussion, it is important to keep in mind that your end goal should not be to ensure that you win out at the expense of anyone else involved, being self-confident doesn't mean always getting your way; it is more about directing the conversation in a way that solves the initial issue in the most effective way possible. This is why it is so important to have a clear idea what it is you are going to say before getting started as you can be sure that you will only get one chance to make a first impression and it is going to set the tone for the entire encounter, guaranteed.

Don't be afraid to fake it

The fact of the matter is that while you can certainly build up your self-confidence over time, you don't need to wait nearly that long in order to reap all of its benefits. While it might seem surprising, consider a conversation with another person both as you would be with confidence and as you would be if you did not have confidence but you were pretending that you did. Now picture both conversations as seen by the other party in the conversation, you should not be surprised to learn that their experience is virtually identical in both scenarios. Essentially what this means is that the best way to appear self-confident is to simply act as you would if you actually had self-confidence.

This will have the added bonus of not only making you appear as though you are more confident to those around you, but also get you in the habit of acting in a self-confident fashion at all times and in all situations. If this seems too good to be true, just give it a try once and you will never again question the results. The positive results from the first interaction can then compound on themselves, making the next interaction even easier and the one after that easier still. Once you find the ability to be confident in the face of adversity you will know that you have the ability to commit to the long-lasting change that you are looking for.

Chapter 4: Changing Personal Patterns

When it comes to setting out down the path to the type of change that you are looking to cultivate, the first thing you will need to consider are the various patterns that you naturally find yourself returning to time, after time, after time. There are patterns everywhere you look, both in your personal behavior and in the behavior of the world as a whole and if you ever hope to see the type of long term changes that will really help you improve yourself, recognizing them as you interact with them is key.

You are in luck once again, however, as much like self-discipline, pattern recognition is a skill which means that it will take you roughly 10,000 hours in order to consider yourself a master of it. This, in turn, means that you are going to need to get started ASAP. You will likely find that the following tips make doing so much easier than it might otherwise be.

See the patterns around you: Before you can get started pointing out your personal patterns, you may find that looking at the patterns of the world around you, helps to put you in the type of mindset that you are looking to cultivate. Once you know what to look for, you will find manmade as well as natural patterns virtually everywhere you look. Look for patterns that repeat anywhere from the leaves on the nearest tree to the cracks in the sidewalk as you walk down the street. After you start attuning to these patterns more regularly, you will then find that more complex and abstract patterns begin to appear as well. This means that you are going to want to try and see the patterns in the behaviors of the people you interact with on a daily basis. Only once you can see all the patterns happening around you at all times and understand how they intersect will you have the knowledge that you need to turn this ability inward and find the patterns that are currently preventing you from reaching the level of change that you seek.

If at first you cannot see the patterns that influence your day, the best place to start is with all of the things that you can currently count on to happen every single day, almost as if they were clockwork. From there you can work backwards and determine why each event happens in the same way every day and so on and so forth until you can accurately determine the cause and effect of everything around you. Don't worry if you can't find all of the information that you need in order to make all the required logical connections, you don't need to make sense of everything immediately, just note the inconsistencies and move on for now. Noticing the patterns is the proper first step in what will eventually be the right direction.

Find patterns for the patterns: After you feel as though you have a fairly detailed grasp on the patterns that are affecting you on a daily basis as well as those that are broadly affecting the world at large, the next step is to take things a step further and consider how all of those various patterns fit together in the most logical way possible. It is especially helpful in this phase to make a point of grouping related patterns into larger groups and looking for further similarities from there. Grouping patterns that are only tangentially related as purely a way of simplifying things for yourself is not recommended however and is likely a good way to skew your data. What's more, you are going to want to leave yourself open to the possibly that once you start looking at the big picture you are going to find something that you missed in the first place which means that you may need to go back and reassess a number of things to ensure you are following the most logical path to success. Before moving on to the next phase it is important that you feel as though you have as clear of a grasp on the big picture as possible as it is the only way you can make truly informed decisions moving forward when it comes to determining how to change most effectively in the shortest period of time possible.

Start looking for patterns to change: Once you have a clear idea of the patterns as they stand, you can start doing your best to determine what should be changed first for the greatest overall result as well as those you want to double down on to ensure they keep happening the way they currently are for as long as possible. Changing personal patterns is easier said than done, however, as it involves changing personal habits as well, some of which may have been in place for an exceedingly long time. Planning is key at this juncture as it will be extremely easy for you to slip up and fall back into your old habits with really even thinking about it.

As an example, imagine that you take on too much work on a regular basis as a way of avoiding deeper human interactions. With this in mind, you could then make a concentrated effort to not work as much on the weekends, and force yourself to follow through by working with coworkers to ensure that the work gets done without requiring extra personal sacrifice on your end.

It is extremely important to follow through on altering the first few patterns that you notice for their negative influence as starting and failing to follow through on personal change is an extremely easy pattern to get into all on its own. If you ever hope to make real progress towards the change that you are aiming for then you need to make sure your pattern regarding change is positive rather than negative. Furthermore, you are going to want to keep in mind the fact that it takes more to making a new plan to change deeply ingrained patterns, it also takes commitment, plenty of time and a state of hyper vigilance that will prevent the pattern from showing up again when you least expect it.

Ideally, the best way to go about changing a specific pattern is to replace it whole cloth with another pattern that is going to fulfil a similar need in a more productive fashion. This new pattern will need to avoid all of the triggers for the old pattern so it may take a while for it to form properly before you get the hang of it. Regardless, it is important to keep it up and not use small instances of failure as an excuse for additional failures further down the line. Remember, it doesn't matter as much if you always stick to the new pattern right away, any variation from the previous pattern can be considered a victory.

Negative patterns: While you are taking stock of the patterns that you most commonly find yourself repeating, it is important to pay special attention to certain negative patterns that are going to make it much more difficult to change for the better than it otherwise might. First and foremost, you are going to want to work to stamp out any patterns that are born from a need for instant gratification as this ideal will only make it more difficult for you to properly commit to long term plans that may lead to a greater degree of overall betterment later on. Furthermore, many people may believe that ignorance is bliss but giving in to patterns that promote ignorance will only lead you to even greater issues further down the line.

Another important pattern to avoid is one that indicates a desire for a strong degree of control over everything around you no matter what. While taking control of your life is an important part of making positive, long-lasting changes, looking for too much control will only ever end in disaster. Another common negative pattern is one that indicates your propensity for flight or fight is skewed too far in on direction or another. Remember, balance is a key to ensuring that this response does not negatively affect your ability to ensure positive change which means you may need to be aware of your gut reaction to conflict and work to rebalance it accordingly.

Positive Patterns: While you are vigorously scouring your psyche for negative patterns to eliminate, it is also important that you keep an eye out for positive habits that are worth focusing on improving as well. Doing so will make it easier to know what types of change will come easily when you get started and what you will need to work on more rigorously moving forward. The most important types of habits to cultivate are those that promote loving yourself, as loving yourself and feeling that you deserve change is an important step to creating lasting progress in the long term. Additionally, you are going to want to keep a sharp eye out for patterns that promote a growth mindset based on expecting positive results to come from positive actions. Finally, other positive patterns to look out for include being aware of personal boundaries and when and where they do not need to be change and also those that promote being more in tune with your personal intuition.

Stinking thinking

While removing negative patterns from your life is going to provide you with numerous benefits in both the short and the long term, they are not the source of the problem. That, in fact, lies with one of the biggest obstacles to true personal change that you will ever encounter: the shadow of negative thoughts. Negative thoughts come in four types and it is important to always be on the lookout for each to prevent them from taking over your thought patterns entirely.

All or nothing thoughts: One of the most common type of negative thoughts are those that make any success seem like failure unless you are absolutely the best of the best, beyond a shadow of a doubt. Known as all or nothing thoughts, they can suck the joy from minor successes and make it more difficult to stay the course to true change, especially when it is going to require hard work and sacrifice to achieve completely. Remember, while everyone likes being the best, the fact of the matter is that a majority of the time the differences between being the best and being quite good at something are relatively minor. Always have a drive for success, just be sure that it is not the only thing that you are focused on otherwise true change will likely never come.

Disqualifying the positives: Another commonly seen type of negative thoughts is what is known as disqualifying the positives. This type of negative thinking occurs when all of the negative possibilities related to a positive course of change converge whenever you look to the future making it impossible for you to see the positive possibilities as well. This type of negative thinking can best be exemplified by the behavior of anyone who has ever generate online content and then focused exclusively on the negative comments they received about it to the point of ignoring the positives entirely. Those who have not yet learned to mitigate these types of habits will find that they have a hard time sticking with change in the long term as it will always inevitably seem futile.

Disqualifying the positives is similar to another type of negative thought known as negative self-labeling. In this instance, you apply socially acceptable labels to yourself to make it easier to avoid making positive changes that will ultimately be more difficult to pursue in the long term. Labels such as emotional, bad at math, or soft touch are all just excuses and treating them as such is the first step to changing them for the better, for good.

Also similar pattern of negative thought is known as projecting which involves taking your own fears related to your shortcomings and placing them onto those around you. These thoughts are then often compounded by a desire to seek the approval of those you meet which is then impossible to achieve because of the projections. The most effective way to fight off these types of thoughts is through the use of if/then statements. Thinking in this binary format will naturally help to motivate you towards change as it provides a clear path from the action in question to the intended result. With an end result in mind you should find that it takes much more force for the negative thoughts to encroach on your change focused mentality.

Chapter 5: Determining Your Goals for the Future

Once you have lain the ground work to ensure that the change you do decide to enact is going to stick, it will be time to consider the goals that you can set to ensure you take advantage of your new mentality as effectively as possible. The best way to go about doing so is through what are known as SMART goals. Simply put, the SMART system posits that all goals should be achievable, specific, measurable, relevant and have a stiff timeline that by and large cannot be changed in order to ensure that the goals you undertake are going to be legitimately worth your time and all of the effort that you plan on exerting making them a reality.

The first SMART goal that you set should be one that is at the same time straightforward enough to more or less ensure your success while at the same time being relevant enough to your day to day life that actually succeeding will be a moment that you can easily recall in the future when success on a future goal is not nearly so assured. This way you will start forming the right type of neural pathways as soon as possible, which will then form into patterns which will eventually become habits. With this in mind you want to start off with a goal that is, at least tangentially connected to the negative pattern that you are the most anxious to start to change. You don't need to have an exact goal in mind at this point, just the start of an idea that you can build into something larger later on. Consider the following to ensure that you are on the right track.

Specificity is key: Good goals are specific which means you want to be sure that the goal you choose is extremely clear, especially when you are first starting out, as goals that are less well defined are much easier to avoid doing in favor of activities that provide more positive stimulation in a shorter period of time. Keeping specific goals in mind will instead make it much easier for you to go ahead and power through whatever task you are currently undertaking.

As an example, consider the goal of getting in shape. While this is certainly a goal that is worth pursuing, if you don't have anything more specific in mind than that, it is unlikely you will ever actually get started because there is simply too much that remains unknown for it to be the type of goal that will actually get you motivated to find the success that you are dreaming of. Rather than "get in shape" a better goal would be to go to the gym at least four times each week as this will provide you with a clear point of success or failure so you always know exactly where you stand when it comes to bringing about the change that you seek.

When you aren't quite sure if the goal you have chosen is specific enough to actually improve your chance of changing for the better, you may be able to figure it out by running through the who, why, where, when and how of the goal. Specifically, you are going to want to consider who is going to be involved with you when it comes to the completion of the goal? What exactly is it that is going to be accomplished? Where the what will be taking place and why it is important that you ensure it is completed as quickly as possible and how exactly you can expect to go about doing it. Once you can answer all five of the big questions then you know you have a goal that is specific enough to generate the type of results that you are looking for.

Easily measured: In addition to being specific, you want the goal that you ultimately land on to be one whose progress can easily be measured as you go along. Not only will this help you to more easily stay on track throughout the entire process, it will make the overall change easier to attain as it will be done in incremental pieces that you can feel good about completing every single time. This incremental process will help allow you to create the types of new neural pathways that you are looking for as they are the first step to creating the types of positive patterns that promote change that you are looking for.

When it comes to doing the actually measuring, the metric that you choose can either be one that is based on achieving specific goals or simply improving time over time, the details don't matter as long as your measurements allow you to clearly determine points for success as well as failure. If you don't have the fear of failure to help motivate you, odds are the going will seem a lot tougher than it otherwise might. As an example, consider the gym example from above, remember it is specific because you have committed to going 4 times a week but if you add the caveat that your end goal is to lose 20 pounds then it will be measurable as well. In order to create a goal that you are sure is measurable, start by determining how you will know that you have met your goal before working backwards from that point. Ideally, you will want to be able to describe your goals in terms of how much or how many.

After you have a clear idea of how you plan to measure your goal, the next thing that you will want to do is determine a way you can externally keep track of your goal, preferably in a visual fashion, as a tool to help you refocus on your success when you become especially tempted to give up the ghost and stray back to your old habits. Visual reminders of all of the hard work that you have put in so far can easily serve as an extremely potent motivator to help you keep at it. If you are working at something that is a bit more esoteric then work out some connection to the physical world that you can make, anything to help encourage you to keep up the good work. Remember, if you are having a hard time remaining committed to a goal and the end seems out of sight, try telling yourself that you only have to push onward until the midpoint as everything else is all going to be downhill.

When it comes to keeping notes of what you are working on, your process for doing so can be anything as simply as a basic line graph or something as detailed as a full scrapbook and journal documenting your experiences. You may need to try multiple types of data collection to see what works for you, but it is important that you keep at it to ensure the best results.

Definitely Attainable: Perhaps more important than anything else, if a goal that you set is unattainable, especially the first goal that you set using this system, then you are going to unknowingly be wasting valuable time and energy while creating negative patterns that end in failure at the same time. What's more, you will end up reinforcing fixed mindset ideals making this a bad choice any way that you look at it. This means that when it comes to setting goals you are going to want to have a clear understanding of your current situation and everything that you currently have going on in your life that will make you less likely to succeed as far as that goal is concerned.

It is important to keep in mind how important it is to assess your situation honestly as the only person you are going to hurt if you sugarcoat things is yourself as you will ultimately end up creating a goal that is unsustainable in the long term. As an example, while exercising at the gym four times a week as a way of ultimately losing twenty pounds might seem realistic on the surface, the fact that you have a job that has you working 80 hours a week, often unexpectedly, can make that goal much less doable than it other might be. When you find a goal that you are enthusiastic about, but that doesn't quite work in its current form, it is important not to give up on it immediately and to instead work to reconstruct it into something that you can actually attain.

Besides taking any time or lifestyle constraints into consideration, you are going to want to be sure that the goal you choose initially is a goal that you are enthusiastic about as it will make it easier to keep up the positive momentum that you start out with once the initial novelty fades and you are forced to get down to the serious work if you ever hope to find the success you seek. When deciding on the overall level of difficulty of the first goal that you set, be sure you are equally as enthusiastic about it for the best results. This is only required at first, eventually you will find that you are able to set your mind to any goal you like regardless of your level of enthusiasm for what you may have to do.

Relevant to your current situation: It is important that the goal you choose is relevant to your current situation as well as being simply something that is attainable with only a reasonable amount of effort. Relevance is key to turning the SMART goal system from a one-time thing into a pattern and eventually a life-long habit that you can rely on to help you meet the challenges of life no matter what they may be. Remember, you want these early goals to be as meaningful as possible so that you think back on them regularly and fortify the neural pathways as quickly as possible so them become your brain's default way of acting.

As an example, consider the fact that even if you set a goal of going to the gym four times each week and then manage to go on to lose twenty pounds, if your level of athleticism or your general weight weren't issues that you had ever given much thought then no new neural pathways will be formed and you risk falling back on negative habits. When it comes to completing your first goal successfully you may find it helpful to break it down into more manageable chunks to start before adding a piece of each chunk to the list of things you need to do each day. If you take it slow you will find that completing part of the task related to achieving your current goal will become habit just like anything else which will thin make it easier to work on even more complicated tasks in turn. As with everything else described above, when working on cementing SMART goals in your life you will want to remember that practice makes perfect.

Create a strict timeline: While you won't be able to tell a proper SMART goal apart from the rest by just looking at a few of its properties, you will always be able to identify one by its strict timetable including a firm start and finish date. Ultimately it will not matter how measurable, specific, relevant and attainable your goal is as without a firm timeframe for you to complete it in, the odds of it actually seeing completion drop below 20 percent.

As an example, consider all the time you have hypothetically been spending at the gym in the previous examples. If you don't set a firm deadline for when you want to finish losing the 20 pounds, you may as well just double down on the snacks instead as it is unlikely you will ever get to where you need to be. Knowing that you have to lose the weight within six months will give you the motivation to power through the moments where sticking to the basics outlined in your weight loss plan seems like more trouble than its worth.

It is important that you don't take from this the fact that no timeline is malleable, as it is perfectly natural for timelines to change as new data regarding the goal is uncovered. The important thing is then to ensure that you are not moving your goals for the wrong reasons and only updating things based on hard facts that previously were only guessed at using anecdotal information. It is important to do as much research as possible before setting a firm goal and then to only change it when it turns out that your initial information is wrong, never for internal reasons related purely to giving yourself more time to goof off and avoid doing what needs to be done.

Once you have a fire deadline in place, the last thing that you will need to do is to determine how to go about getting from where you are now to where you ultimately want to be at the deadline. Returning once again to the weight loss example, in order to lose twenty pounds in six months you only need to lose three pounds per week, and keep it off, which is a goal that almost anyone can hit with the proper amount of hard work and dedication. Setting these benchmarks will not only give you a clear idea of whether or not your goal is realistic, it will help you know exactly what you need to do each week in order to get to where you need to be. Even better, it will make the whole process seem more manageable because you won't be thinking about the end result all at once and instead be focused on several smaller goals instead.

Conclusion

Thank for making it through to the end of *The Power of Habits Change your thoughts change your life live in happiness*, let's hope it was informative and able to provide you with all of the tools you need to achieve your goals whatever it is that they may be. Just because you've finished this book doesn't mean there is nothing left to learn on the topic, expanding your horizons is the only way to find the mastery you seek.

The next step is to stop reading already and to get ready to prepare yourself to make the sorts of major life changes that you have been putting off for far too long. Remember, it doesn't matter how far-fetched the long-term changes that you want to make may seem right now, if you break it down into realistic chunks them you will be surprised at how quickly you can actually turn your dreams into reality. While the first goal that you are planning to set might not seem like much at the moment, the truth of the matter is that it is akin to the acorn that can grow into the mighty oak tree. If you persevere now and see your first goal through to the end, then that will start to create the types of neural pathways that will eventually lead to positive patterns and positive habits that could very well last the rest of your life.

While you may be tempted to skip over the small changes and jump right to the major, life changing alterations, it is important to start small rather than risk overextending early on and hurting your chances of trying again a second time without a fixed mindset taking over. Overall it is often best to think of change as a marathon, not a sprint, slow and steady wins the race. Continue putting one foot in front of the other and you can see real change before you know it.

Finally, if you found this book useful in anyway, a review on Amazon is always appreciated!

About the Author

Thomas Garry is a passionate entrepreneur, author, and motivational speaker who currently resides in Perth, Western Australia.

Starting out, Thomas worked as a salesman in the technology industry and dabbled in network marketing. After years of extensive studying and soul-searching, he decided to work for himself and become an entrepreneur. Nearly a decade later, Thomas had to make the difficult decision to close his company. This failure ultimately served as his driving force.

Today, Thomas is infinitely dedicated to providing people with the tools necessary to unleash their limitless potential so that they can achieve their goals. Through his motivational methods, he teaches others to face challenges head on so that they can finally live the life that they have always dreamed of.

Thomas Garry has been happily married for 20 years and is the proud father of two sons.

"Nothing binds you except your thoughts; nothing limits you except your fear; and nothing controls you except your beliefs. Everything is within you."
-Marianne Williamson

www.ingramcontent.com/pod-product-compliance
Lightning Source LLC
Chambersburg PA
CBHW051259170526
45165CB00004B/1777